GOOD YONI

Natural Cures for Feminine Health

BY NIKKI LOVE

DEDICATIONS

This book is dedicated to my late Mother Phyllis Harris, who instilled the gift of writing inside of me, who loved me unconditionally, who taught me self-care, who exemplified divine femininity. I love you and miss you dearly.

Special thanks to the love of my life London Thomas, who brings out the best in me, who embraces the Goddess in me and who loves me completely and entirely. Thank you for your unconditional love and support. I love you for eternity.

TABLE OF CONTENTS

INTRODUCTION

Yoni is Sanskrit for the female genitalia, the womb, vulva, female energy, divine creation or simply, the vagina. The Yoni is the gateway of all births, it is essential for life, love and happiness. It is the source and the origin of life. Life would cease to exist without it. It is the very essence of physical pleasure.

The Yoni is power! It is the most powerful force that moves through the entire universe. The Yoni is the most important part of the female body. There are natural ways to restore, rejuvenate, prevent and heal disease and other ailments common to the female reproductive system. Good yoni is a healthy yoni.

Good yoni health is based on several factors; age, diet, genetics, hormones, personal habits, hygiene and mental health. They are all connected. The Yoni not only represents the physical aspect of the body but also the emotional and psychological.

As a woman ages her estrogen levels decrease, this can cause a variety of health concerns including irregular cycles and infertility. Low estrogen can also cause vaginal dryness and painful intercourse. On the contrast, xenoestrogens from plastics, cosmetics and food preservatives can mimic natural estrogen which can cause fibroids, uterine cancers, endometriosis, ovarian cysts and breast tumors. Hormones should be properly balanced for optimal yoni health.

The ph of your yoni is very important. Diet, personal habits, sexual habits and certain products can alter the ph of the yoni causing inflammation, infections and unpleasant odors. The normal ph of the yoni is somewhere between 3.8 – 4.5. If the normal ph balance is altered, the natural environment can be disrupted and sets the stage for bad bacteria. Menstruation and hormone fluctuations can also disrupt the normal ph of the yoni.

The yoni if often referred to as "self-cleaning". A healthy yoni is colonized by naturally occurring flora, microorganisms present to fight off infections and maintain a healthy flow of self-cleaning discharge.

Every woman is different, not all women have the proper balance of normal vaginal flora to keep this mechanism working. Vaginal flora is largely dependent upon gut flora to keep the female ecosystem in balance.

Overuse of antibiotics can destroy good bacteria needed to keep the body and the yoni healthy. An overall balance of good bacteria is essential to yoni health.

Physical health determines your yoni health. Medical issues, chronic conditions, disease, toxins and those under medical treatment may experience symptoms of vaginal discomfort such as itching and burning. Treating underlying health problems will greatly improve your yoni's natural environment and holistic well-being.

The yoni is sacred. It is valued. It is honored and cherished. A woman's mental health towards her body is important. Poor psychological well-being can negatively impact your yoni.

Stress, depression and anxiety can cause vaginal dryness or abnormal discharge, apathy towards sex, painful intercourse and other reproductive issues.

Your yoni is divine it should be praised, respected and revered. Through awareness and consciousness learn to love your yoni, perform self-care rituals, be self-confident, and realize its power and its purpose. Practice yoni care daily by nourishing, cleansing, purifying and accepting it as your own personal sanctuary.

This book will give you simple home remedies for your Yoni with natural substances some dating as far back as 2000 years ago. Healing the Yoni can be achieved by educating yourself and dedicating your time to pampering yourself, loving your womanhood, adopting a healthy lifestyle, cultivating your divine feminine energy and most of all loving the goddess that lives within you!

BALANCING HORMONES

Hormones are secreted from the glands of the endocrine system then enter into the bloodstream. Each gland has a specific function that affects different organs in the body. Most bodily functions are regulated by hormones. Hormones are chemical messengers so to speak, they send signals that tell your body what to do and when to do it. If there is too much or too little hormone in the bloodstream there is an imbalance. There are several hormones in the human body but there are 5 main female hormones that affect the reproductive system:

- Estrogen – is a female sex hormone. Estrogen helps breasts and uterine lining grow, controls libido and sexual fluids, balances cholesterol, blood sugar, and controls mood and memory.

- Progesterone – is a female sex hormone. Progesterone helps the body prepare for pregnancy and controls menstrual cycles.

- Testosterone – is a steroid hormone that is predominantly a male sex hormone but is produced in women in small amounts. Testosterone controls libido, cognitive function, energy, and bone and muscle mass.

- Luteinizing Hormone – controls the reproductive system. This hormone is what causes the ovaries to release an egg during ovulation.

- Follicle Stimulating Hormone – is produced in both men

and women. In women it releases eggs, in men it makes sperm. FSH helps maintain menstrual cycles.

It is common for women to be unbalanced in estrogen and progesterone. As a woman ages, her estrogen levels drop resulting in menopause. After childbirth, estrogen levels also drop. Low levels of estrogen in pre-menopausal women often result in female reproductive problems.

When the body has too much estrogen and not enough progesterone, this is called estrogen dominance. Excess estrogen can cause a wide range of conditions including PMS, fatigue, infertility, endometriosis, fibroids, fibrocystic breasts, decreased libido and certain cancers, especially breast cancer. On the flip side, excess progesterone causes low energy, weight gain, depression, headaches, skin problems and other side effects.

It is natural for hormones to fluctuate at times (such as after your menstrual cycle) but they can also be affected by environmental endocrine disruptors (industrial chemicals, preservatives, cosmetics, food, etc.) or certain medical conditions. It is important to get your hormone levels checked by a trained professional. Take special care to make sure your hormones are properly balanced for optimal yoni health and overall health and well-being.

Causes of hormonal imbalances include:

- Stress
- Weight Gain
- Poor Diet
- Birth Control
- Underactive or Overactive Thyroid

- Type 1 and 2 Diabetes
- Cancer and certain infections
- Iodine Deficiency
- Xenoestrogens (found in chemicals, toxins, pesticides)
- PCOS (polycystic ovary syndrome)
- Menopause

Symptoms of hormonal imbalances:

- Irregular or painful periods
- Abnormal uterine bleeding
- Vaginal atrophy (Dryness)
- Hot flashes
- Night sweats
- Infertility
- Hair growth on face, neck or back
- Reduced sex drive
- Breast tenderness
- Bloating
- Changes in appetite

Natural remedies for balancing hormones:

Diet is the foundation that helps to balance your hormones. A healthy diet should include whole foods, organic foods, unprocessed foods and organic meats with no growth hormones. Try adopting a plant based diet.

Sugar, flour, dairy and gluten can trigger hormonal imbalances by causing inflammation. Most people are not aware of allergies or sensitivity to wheat products. Gluten can cause leaky gut and other problems that contribute to hormonal imbalances.

Try gluten-free foods when possible.

Dairy products often contain growth hormones and antibiotics that contribute to hormone imbalances. Animal products have high amounts of hormones. Cut back on fatty meats, cheese, milk etc. Try plant or nut milks instead of cow's milk.

- Drink plenty of clean filtered water
- Eat lots of veggies and fresh fruit
- Consume herbs and herbal teas
- Eat foods with natural sources of estrogen such as:
  o Flaxseed
  o Almonds, peanuts, pistachios
  o Chickpeas, red beans, black beans, black-eyed peas, green peas, split peas
  o Tofu, miso, tempeh
  o Olives and olive oil
  o Dry fruits

Omega-3 fatty acids support the construction of hormones and regulate important bodily functions. Omega-3 fatty acids are not naturally produced by the body; therefore, they must be acquired through diet or supplementation. Fish oil & Cod liver oil is a great source of Omega-3 fatty acids.

Magnesium relaxes the central nervous system, reduces inflammation and prevents excess cortisol (stress hormone), all of which are needed to balance hormones.

Vitamin D is a hormone that boosts the immune system and boosts levels of estrogen and progesterone.

B Complex boosts progesterone and works with your liver to remove excess estrogen from the body.

Maca Root (Peruvian Ginseng) is an endocrine regulator that contains nutrients necessary to support hormonal imbalance. It is good for infertility and improves sexual functions.

Chaste berry(Vitex) supports your pituitary gland to produce progesterone and luteinizing hormone which are necessary for regular menstrual cycles and hormones. It is also a great tool for infertility and regular ovulation.

Probiotics supports the gut microbiome that produces the enzyme that supports the metabolization of estrogen and helps guide hormones from the body.

Green Tea contains Theanine, a compound that reduces the release of the stress hormone cortisol. It also contains antioxidants that lower the risk of disease.

Exercise increases the levels of human growth hormone (Hgh) and testosterone. Exercise also balances progesterone and reduces levels of insulin (fat hormone).

Reduce Stress hormones cortisol, adrenaline and norepinephrine, the three stress hormones commonly known as the "fight or flight" system. High levels of these hormones can make you more prone to infections and disease. Learn relaxation techniques such as yoga and meditation, laugh more and practice mindfulness.

Proper Rest increases Melatonin, the hormone released by the pineal gland. It is responsible for regulating your sleep cycle. It also is responsible for regulating your menstrual cycle. Therefore, sleep is paramount in keeping your hormones in proper balance.

Stop Smoking to rebalance your hormones. The chemicals in cigarette smoke cause disease and degeneration in the body. Smoking disrupts the endocrine system which contributes to reproductive disease, menstrual problems, infertility and early menopause.

Detoxing will eliminate toxins and excess estrogen. Try a liver cleanse, intermittent fasting, or a lemon juice and baking soda. Juice cleanses for 10 days or more has been proven to eliminate toxins from the body. Take Chlorophyll, Activated Charcoal, and/or Diatomaceous Earth for extra cleansing.

HEALING YONI DRYNESS
(VAGINAL ATROPHY)

Yoni dryness can be caused by low estrogen levels, most common in women after menopause; however, atrophy can happen to any woman at any age due to underlying issues including low estrogen, certain medications, or illness.

Natural lubrication from the cervix travels down the vagina to cleanse and remove dead cells keeping the yoni healthy. The Bartholins Gland of the yoni produces extra moisture during sexual excitement to keep the yoni supple and protect the vaginal walls. At times the Bartholins Gland can get blocked by small cysts resulting in vaginal atrophy. Treatment for Bartholins cysts require surgery if the cyst does not rupture on its own. Other treatments include sitz baths and anti-inflammatory medication.

A dry yoni does not only affect you as a woman but it is very painful for your partner during sex due to friction and burning of the skin. Good yoni is not a dry yoni. Here are a few natural ways to heal yoni dryness:

Foreplay is very important in warming the yoni up and giving the Bartholins Gland time to produce sufficient lubrication. Try tantric sex, meditating together, and creating a romantic atmosphere with candles and essential oils. Wake up the senses and allow your natural energy to flow.

Coconut Oil is a great lubricant for yoni dryness. It also has antibacterial, antimicrobial and antiviral properties, so it can prevent infections during sex. Lubricate your lady parts by adding coconut oil to your daily diet. Coconut oil can be taken internally, or it can be placed inside of the yoni.

Aloe Vera is rich in vitamins and minerals that hydrate and relieve irritations. It gives a protective barrier and heals the skin by increasing natural collagen. Aloe can lubricate the yoni due to its ability to draw in moisture. It has astringent properties and penetrates into the deepest layers of skin. Aloe Vera is a miracle for the yoni. It keeps it young, supple and fresh the natural way. Using Aloe Vera from natural plants is always best. Try to avoid products with chemicals or preservatives. Aloes can be taken internally and applied inside of the yoni.

Seabuckthorne Fruit Oil is the richest source of Omega - 7. It contains Palmitoleic Acid that has been used in ancient medicinal practices for replenishing natural skin oils and increasing vaginal moisture. Apply to the inside and outside of the yoni to regenerate epithelial cells. Use after sex to prevent UTI's as Seabuckthorne oil prevents the overgrowth of E. Coli. It can offer protection from herpes and HIV as well. Use Seabuckthorne oil internally and as a sexual lubricant.

Macadamia Nuts are also a natural source of Omega 7, which hydrates the mucous membrane. It helps to alleviate dry yoni tissues and improve the vaginal lining and elasticity. You can also take Macadamia Nut oil internally for good results.

Vitamin E Oil contains Tocopheryl which assists in cellular skin restoration and healing. Taken internally, it increases blood supply to yoni tissues. Vitamin E is an antioxidant which fights off free radicals on the skin and helps prevent the skin from damage. It is touted as one of the most effective moisturizers. Use Vitamin E oil capsules internally as a dietary supplement or apply directly to your yoni.

Hyaluronic Acid is a naturally occurring substance produced by the body. It is a gel-like water binding molecule that helps lubricate the skin. Hyaluronic Acid can be used cosmetically but you can also get it from certain foods such as:

o   Bone broth
o   White & Sweet potatoes,
o   Kale
o   Dark chocolate
o   Red meat
o   Almonds
o   Red wine
o   Citrus fruits

Water is a simple remedy for yoni dryness. Most women are severely dehydrated. Our bodies are made up of 70% water. Water lubricates cells, joints, organs, muscles and tissues making it essential to health. Drinking 8 to 10 glasses of water a day can revitalize your yoni.

Alcohol can dehydrate your yoni tissues due to its diuretic effects. Alcohol removes fluids from your body at a faster rate than normal. If you drink alcoholic beverages, be sure to drink plenty of water or electrolyte beverages to prevent dehydration.

TIGHTENING THE YONI

Over time with age and through childbirth, the muscles of the yoni become less elastic and the pelvic floor becomes weaker. Lack of movement or exercise can also make the pelvic region weak. Researchers say that frequent sex can't make the yoni loose, but it doesn't take a rocket scientist to figure that one out. Even shoes stretch after wearing them for awhile! Let's take a look at some natural ways to tighten the yoni:

Yoni Eggs are small egg shaped semiprecious stones used to strengthen the pelvic floor, enhance sexual experience (better orgasms), tone the bladder, increase blood flow to the uterus, and promote feminine energy. Crystal yoni eggs can bring spiritual and emotional healing due to their vibrational frequency. Jade, Clear Quartz or Rose Quartz yoni eggs have the best healing properties. Yoni eggs come in different sizes, the larger eggs should be used first, and then the smaller eggs as your muscles tighten over a period of time. You can also use yoni eggs during meditation and sexual intercourse for a more powerful experience.

Ben Wa Balls are similar to yoni eggs with the purpose of strengthening the pelvic floor and vaginal muscles. The difference is that Ben Wa balls are shaped like a marble with a small weight inside. They are traditionally used to enhance sexual and orgasmic experience.

Kegel exercises are often prescribed by practitioners for tightening the yoni. It involves squeezing and releasing your pelvic muscles repeatedly for a specific amount of time. Kegels can be practiced anywhere, on the toilet, in the car or at your desk at work.

Certain products can be used internally to tighten the yoni. Some can only be temporary while others can take months to see results. Take care to check ingredients on products before inserting them into your yoni as some can cause allergic reactions or infections.

Alum also called potassium alum is used in baking powders, cosmetics and medicines. It is widely known for its skin tightening properties. It is used in sexual health products for shrinking the tissues of the yoni. Alum provides temporary tightening lasting up to 1 hour. It is best used right before sex. Dissolve Alum in warm water and insert vaginally using a vaginal applicator. Always apply natural oil after using Alum to prevent dryness.

Manjakani also called Oak Galls, is popular in India and Malaysia. It has been used after childbirth for ages. It is rich in vitamins, tannins and gallic acid. It also has antimicrobial and anti-inflammatory properties. Manjakani tightens yoni muscles, reduces discharge, tightens skin and sagging breasts, and removes unpleasant yoni odors.

Kacip Fatimah is a healing plant used for the female reproductive system. It contains phytoestrogens that help with healing the vaginal tract. In addition, it balances hormones, increases libido, and lubricates the yoni. Kacip Fatimah + Manjakani will have your yoni tighter in no time.

Shatavari in Hindu means "having 100 spouses". It is an Ayurvedic herb that has been used for 5000 years. It is a medicinal plant that contains vitamins and phytoestrogens that regulate hormonal secretions. Yes, it makes your yoni wetter. Shatavari is also antibacterial and antifungal meaning it can prevent UTI's and BV.

Curcuma Cumosa belongs to the Turmeric family. It has been used traditionally in Thailand for healing the female genitalia. It tightens and strengthens the vaginal walls, uterus and pelvic muscles. It also prevents the vaginal walls from prolapsing.

Black Cohosh is one of the best home remedies and all natural substances for tightening the yoni. Black Cohosh is a plant that has phytoestrogenic properties. It has been scientifically shown to improve yoni rejuvenation.

Yoni Tightening Wand is an electronic device that uses red and blue laser LED beams to stimulate and heal yoni tissues. It is said to tighten the yoni, eliminate bacteria, heal cervical erosion, detoxify the yoni, treat stress incontinence and enhance sexual sensitivity.

Jamu Stick is an herbal stick designed to be inserted into the yoni to cleanse, tighten, remove deal cells, reduce discharge, and restore vaginal flora. It also has ingredients such as Longjack to increase sexual pleasure. It is made with Manjakani, Jati Belanda, Bolus Alba, Parameria Laevigata, Piper Betle and Alum.

HEALING FIBROIDS, ENDOMETRIOSIS AND PCOS

Fibroids are benign tumors on the uterus. They are made up of fibrous connective tissue that can vary in sizes. 70% - 80% of all women will develop fibroids during the reproductive years when estrogen levels are higher. Recent studies show a link between fibroids and Vitamin D deficiency. Fake estrogens in food, chemicals and beauty products (such as perms and hair dyes) can also encourage fibroids to grow. Complications can range from excessive bleeding to fatigue, back pain and abdominal pain. In serious cases, a hysterectomy (removal of the uterus) may need to be performed. To avoid surgery try these natural remedies:

Green Tea Extract contains the antioxidant called epigallacatechin-gallate (EGCG). It has been shown to shrink fibroids and reduce symptoms. Green tea is full of health benefits for the feminine woman. It is safe to consume every day and has no side effects.

Sheep Sorrell is a perennial herb grown around the world and is traditionally used as medicine. It is known for its use in destroying tumors (cancerous and non-cancerous). It has vitamins and has one of the most potent antioxidants herbs recognized. Sheep Sorrell purifies the blood and dissolves tumors and destroys infectious tissues. It is highly recommended for fibroids.

Blackstrap Molasses is an extraction from raw sugar cane. It contains essential vitamins and minerals which are beneficial for uterine health. Blackstrap Molasses is an age old home remedy for uterine fibroids, PMS and heavy menstrual cycles.

Apple Cider Vinegar alkalizes the body by raising the ph levels when taken internally. ACV also removes toxins from the body which is necessary for healing. ACV baths are particularly helpful in detoxing the yoni and the womb. ACV + Blackstrap Molasses creates a powerful home remedy for uterine fibroids.

Black Seed Oil also called Nigella Sativa contains thymoquinone which is a powerful anticancer, antioxidant that improves the immune system. Black seed oil can help shrink tumors among a host of other diseases. Take oil internally as well as apply as a poultice to the uterus as needed.

Castor Oil packs have been used in medicine for thousands of years. It is high in ricinoleic acid which is antiviral, antibacterial and antifungal. Castor oil is a healing oil that can be applied to the uterus using a flannel cloth and heating pad. Castor oil can also be applied inside the yoni to assist in dissolving cervical tumors.

Witch Hazel *Hamamelis Virginiana* contains a certain tannin called Hamamelitannin which can reduce tumors. The leaves of witch hazel can be made into a tea to drink or the bark can be used to make a poultice to be applied to the uterus.

Karela *Bitter Gourd* is native to India. It is a bitter melon that resembles a cucumber. Karela is packed with vitamins and utrients and is an excellent blood purifier. It detoxifies the kidneys, liver, lungs and digestive tract. The antioxidants in Karela reduce tumors of the breast and cervix. Women have successfully expelled fibroids with Karela.

Vitamin D Studies show that there is connection between women with fibroids and a deficiency in Vitamin D. Get more sun shine and add Vitamin D supplements to your diet. Do not take Vitamin D in large doses or for extended periods of time as it can be toxic.

Flaxseeds remove excess estrogen from the body that make fibroids grow larger. Flaxseeds contain Lignans, a plant compound that have antioxidant properties. Lignans reduce the risk of cancer and abnormal growths. Flaxseeds can be consumed in ground or whole seeds or oil. Combining Flaxseeds with L-Lysine can reduce fibroid tumors in the body.

Eliminating Diet is the most important change you can make that help reduce fibroid growth. What you put in your body is what manifests. Fast foods, junk foods, heavy meat, processed foods, sugars, excess salt, dairy and wheat can clog your cellular energies, and alter your DNA resulting in tumors and other abnormal growths. Some helpful changes in your diet include:

- o   Avoid meats with growth hormones
- o   Avoid undercooked meats
- o   Eat fish and salmon
- o   Eat fresh fruits and vegetables
- o   Eat a plant based diet
- o   Consume beetroot juice
- o   Consume herbal infusions
- o   Eat more fiber
- o   Avoid sugar

- Cut out all dairy products
- Avoid soy products
- Limit alcohol
- Quit smoking

ENDOMETRIOSIS

Endometriosis occurs when the tissue that lines the inside of the uterus begins to grow on the outside of the uterus. It usually affects the ovaries, bowels and pelvic tissues. This scar tissue has no way to exit the body which causes problems such as painful periods, painful sex, infertility, inflammation and bowel/bladder pain. The exact cause of endometriosis in not known, however, it can be healed. Natural remedies for endometriosis include:

Eliminating Diet is beneficial when it comes to healing endometriosis. Studies indicate a higher risk in women with Celiac Disease, an allergic response to gluten. Removing gluten from your diet will improve symptoms. Try gluten-free breads, pastas, and cereals. Avoid soy as well as sugar.

Lycopene is a powerful antioxidant found in fruits and vegetables. It is found in watermelons, tomatoes, grapefruits, papayas and guavas. Lycopene has been sighted as a treatment for dissolving growths and protecting the body from cellular damage. It interrupts the pathway that causes tumors and scar tissue to grow. It is also effective against yeast.

Turmeric is a spice that contains Curcumin, which helps fight foreign invaders in the body, reduces inflammation and repairs cellular damage. It has been shown to inhibit abnormal growths. Turmeric is best take with black or red pepper for best absorption.

Serrapeptase is an enzyme found in silkworms. It reduces inflammation and pain and breaks down dead or damaged tissues. Women who have taken serrapeptase have been reported to have healed endometriosis. It should not be taken with blood thinners, turmeric, garlic or fish oil.

Coptis also called Goldthread is a traditional Chinese herb that is said to enhance overall health. It is a potent anti-inflammatory agent. It is also known for stopping abnormal cell growth and treating parasites. Do not use if pregnant.

Pine Bark Extract is a medicinal herb that contains Pycnogenol. It is a potent antioxidant that is effective in reducing menstrual disorders. It also relieves symptoms of menopause and improves blood circulation.

Endometriosis has been thought to be caused by parasites, although research has not confirmed this claim. Parasites are harmful microorganisms that contaminate the body and feed off internal organs. When parasites feed on the uterus, excess tissue is left behind. Over 50% of the human population is said to carry some kind of parasite in the body. Parasites can hide in places that are not easily detected (such as the outside of the uterus). It is very beneficial to cleanse the body of parasites to encourage healing. Natural ways to get rid of parasites include:

Garlic Capsules will loosen the parasites which makes it easier for them to exit the body.

Diatomaceous Earth is made from fossilized remains of tiny diatoms and is naturally extracted from the earth. It is often used as an insecticide. It causes parasites to die by absorbing fats and oils from them, causing them to dry out. They are carried from the body and flush out through the digestive system. Use food grade diatomaceous earth only.

Bentonite Clay consists of aged volcanic ash. It removes toxins, impurities, chemicals, heavy metals and parasites. It is a great detoxifying agent that kills bacteria and infections. It can be used internally as well as in poultices applied to the abdomen. Use food grade clay only.

POLYCYSTIC OVARY SYNDROME

Polycystic Ovary Syndrome (PCOS) is a hormonal imbalance that causes large ovaries with cysts on them. It causes menstrual irregularities, acne, excessive hair growth, pain, bloating and infertility. PCOS is thought to occur when the pancreas produces too much insulin increasing the androgen hormone including testosterone. This causes abnormal ovulation and when you don't ovulate regularly, it causes negative side effects on the body. PCOS is also a result of low progesterone. Natural remedies for PCOS include:

White Peony Tea is known for its powerful antioxidant benefits. It contains polyphenols that are effective in preventing the mutation of genetic cells and destroys mutated cells. White Peony also reduces insulin levels, which contributes to PCOS.

Chaste berry (Vitex) has been used with success in treating those with PCOS. It normalizes progesterone levels and it suppresses the formation of ovarian cysts.

Iodine is a chemical element that is essential in regulating the thyroid hormones. Low levels of iodine can result in PCOS. Increase your intake of Iodine to help heal PCOS. Natural foods that increase iodine include:

- o Kelp
- o Kombucha
- o Seafood

- Eggs
- Sea Salt
- Pink Himalayan Salt
- Iodine drops

Other foods that increase progesterone:

- Beans
- Cabbage
- Pumpkin
- Brussels sprouts
- Broccoli
- Kale
- Cauliflower
- Nuts and seeds
- Dark Chocolate
- Avocados
- Salmon
- Carrots

HEALING MENORRHAGIA
(HEAVY MENSTRUAL BLEEDING)

Menorrhagia is a condition in which a woman experiences abnormally heavy bleeding during menstruation. Heavy blood loss can cause extreme cramping and anemia. Causes include conditions ranging from fibroids to hormonal imbalances to certain types of birth control. Menorrhagia can affect the quality of life including missing time from work, travel and activities. Natural remedies for Menorrhagia include:

Cayenne Pepper contains Capsicum from a plant used to make medicine. It improves poor circulation and decreases pain associated with menstrual cramps.

Red Raspberry Leaf is the leaf that grows raspberries. It includes the polyphenol called Fragarine, which is known for tightening and toning the muscles in the pelvis, and strengthening the uterus to correct irregular bleeding.

Shepherd's Purse is a plant used in herbal medicine. It contains Fumaric acid and Sulforaphane, which are substances that reduce inflammation, reduces or stops heavy menstrual bleeding and slows the growth of tumors. It can also heal PMS, cramps and UTI's.

Lady's Mantle is a healing plant used to ease aches and pains associated with menstruation. It has astringent properties that tighten and tone uterine tissues. It is very healing to the body and has a positive effect on hormones. Use with Shepherd's Purse for a uterine healing tea.

Yarrow is a healing plant that has been used for thousands of years. It stops excessive blood flow, eases menstrual cramps, reduces pain and inflammation and it relieves congestion of the uterus

Sage is high in nutrients, vitamins and antioxidants that are nourishing to the uterus. Sage balances hormones by naturally increasing estrogen. Drinking Sage tea several times a day can decrease blood flow during menstruation.

Cinnamon Bark has been used for heavy bleeding for ages. Cinnamon bark also reduces insulin resistance in women with PCOS and type 2 Diabetes. Cinnamon Bark can be added to most food and drinks.

Agrimony is a flowering herb that has anticoagulant properties. It is an astringent herb that helps to stop both internal and external bleeding. Agrimony helps to curb menstrual bleeding. Drink as a tea.

Cramp Bark is a plant used for medicine. It has many healing properties, but it is widely known for reducing menstrual bleeding and painful cramps. It is a natural muscle relaxer, sedative and antispasmodic. Cramp Bark strengthens, tones and tightens uterine tissue by constricting blood flow in the body.

MENSTRUAL CYCLES

W omen often feel resentment and hatred towards their period. From the puberty stage, menstruation was seen as dirty, taboo, unclean, sinful and such as punishment or a curse. However, women should love and embrace the fact that their bodies are incredible and amazingly created to give life. Blood is life. Your cycle reflects the phase of creation, over and over and over again. You could not birth such beautiful babies without it.

Most women feel negatively about menstruation because it disrupts the flow of everyday life, the bleeding, the cramps, no sex, fatigue, mood swings etc. Yet we lack true understanding about its design. In certain cultures, menstruation is seen as empowering. It has long been associated with the waxing and waning of the moon. The Egyptians and other indigenous people of the lands celebrated menstruation with ceremonies. I am not saying celebrate your monthly cycle with food and drinks, I'm saying have a different mindset when it comes to your body. What you think about yourself, including your cycle is what manifests in reality.

If you dread your period, hate your time of the month, and resent your womanhood, your cycles will be a reflection of just that. I have personally known women who control their menstrual cycles to little or no bleeding at all. What you put in your body has a great affect on your cycle. Eating meat causes heavy bleeding. Women who eat plant based diets have lighter cycles. Fasting decreases your cycle time, flow and length of time. Women who fast often have lighter cycles as well.

Harboring past trauma, pain, hatred and unforgiveness can cause heavy, painful periods. Stress and bad relationships can cause harsh periods. Learn your body. Love your body. Learn how to nourish your womb. Cleanse your spirit, release anger and bitterness, let go of things that no longer serve you. Eat healthy, drink water, fast, meditate, pray, hang out in nature. Do whatever is necessary to heal your womb. Your womb is your Wombmanhood. If you desire a difference you must make a difference. All women are beautiful inside and out, and you are a divine goddess. Embrace yourself completely. Period and all!

HEALING INFECTIONS

Your yoni creates its own environment from the normal bacteria it produces, called vaginal flora. The main good bacterium is called lactobacilli. Lactobacilli provide protection against microbes by producing lactic acid and hydrogen peroxide which helps maintain a healthy and normal ph. Hydrogen Peroxide prevents the overgrowth of bad bacteria that causes infection. When the lactobacilli levels are disrupted, the flora becomes unbalanced and causes infections such as Bacterial Vaginosis, Candida (Yeast), Cervicitis and Vaginitis. Natural remedies for infections of the yoni:

Candida Albicans is a fungus that naturally lives in your yoni. If there is an overgrowth of Candida it will result in a yeast infection causing itching, pain, burning, discharge and inflammation. Over 75% of women will experience a yeast infection during their lifetime. Candida can also spread to other parts of the body or the bloodstream. Excess use of sugar and antibiotics can create an environment for yeast to grow. Natural treatments for yeast include:

- o   Apple Cider Vinegar
- o   Coconut Oil
- o   Oil of Oregano
- o   Probiotics or Greek Yogurt
- o   Garlic
- o   Tea Tree Oil

- o Wormwood
- o Candida Cleanse
- o Caprylic Acid
- o Do NOT use Boric Acid – it is poisonous

Bacterial Vaginosis is colonized by the microbe Garderella Vaginalis. It occurs when the vaginal flora is disrupted and the ph balance is thrown off. BV is commonly found in sexually active women. The risk of infection increases with multiple sex partners. Natural remedies for BV:

Colloidal Silver is a solution made of silver particles. It has been used in ancient medicine to heal bacterial, fungal and viral infections. It can be used orally and intravaginally.

Hydrogen Peroxide has a ph of about 3.5, the same as a normal healthy yoni. Lactobacilli in the vagina produce hydrogen peroxide that wards off infections. Use Hydrogen Peroxide mixed with equal parts water to relieve symptoms of BV.

Povidone – Iodine is an antiseptic used for skin infections. It has long been used by surgeons to prevent infections during surgery. Povidone – Iodine douches are sold over the counter as "medicated" douches. Povidone – Iodine has been shown to reduce symptoms of BV while recovering good bacteria Lactobacilli. Do not use if sensitive or allergic to Iodine or Shellfish.

Calendula is a plant used for medicine. It has antibacterial, antifungal, anti-inflammatory and antiseptic properties. Studies show it is just as successful in treating BV as Metronidazole. It can also treat yeast infections. Calendula can reach infections of the gut whereas localized treatment cannot. Calendula can be used in oil form, in creams, in herbal tincture or tea.

Other remedies for BV:

- Apple Cider Vinegar
- Probiotics
- Tea Tree Oil suppositories
- Mega doses of Vitamin B Complex

HPV (Human Papilloma Virus) – Is the most common sexually transmitted disease in the US. It is a virus that is spread by having oral, vaginal or anal sex with someone who carries the virus. Genital warts are a sign of HPV. Some women do not have symptoms until cervical cancer surfaces. Sometimes HPV will go away on its own within 2 years of infection, but in other cases HPV infection can develop into cancers of the vagina, mouth or anus. There is a natural way to cleanse HPV virus from the body:

Make a mixture of Colloidal Silver, Tea Tree Oil and Oregano Oil

- Colloidal Silver 4 oz
- Tea Tree Oil 1 oz
- Oregano Oil ½ oz.

Mix together in a small plastic bottle. Use 1 vaginal applicator full of mixture at bedtime for 7 days. Also, orally consume Colloidal Silver and Oregano Oil daily for 14 days to eradicate HPV in the mouth, esophagus and stomach. Women have reported to heal HPV with this remedy.

Cervical Erosion occurs when the cells inside your cervix begin to grow on the outside. It can cause bleeding between periods and after sex. It also causes excessive discharge. Cervical erosion can be caused by hormones, pregnancy, birth control or ertain infections. Cervical erosion often goes away on its own sometimes it does not. Therapy includes burning or freezing the cells from your cervix. However, you can use Silver Nitrate as a douche to treat cervical erosion naturally.

Cystitis *Urinary Tract Infection* is caused by bacteria that travel to the bladder through the urethra (bladder opening). The most common bacteria found in UTI's is E. Coli, a bacteria that normally lives in the large intestine but eventually works its way into the urethra. One out of five women around the world will acquire a UTI at some point in their lives. Contributing factors are frequent sex (where bacteria can spread from the anus to the yoni), improper cleaning, not emptying the bladder promptly and certain illnesses. The preferred method of treatment is a wide spectrum of antibiotics. Some antibiotics have become resistant to E. Coli, which easily returns to the bladder seen in recurrent infections. If untreated, UTI's can eventually spread to the kidneys and the bloodstream and can cause sepsis which can be fatal. If you have frequent or recurring UTI's it is best to keep them from returning by preventing them. Natural remedies for UTI's:

Cranberry can be taken in pill form or juice, however, pure Cranberry juice with no additives or sugars are best. The active compound, proanthocyanidins helps to prevent bacteria from attaching to the bladder wall. Cranberry pills contain more of this active ingredient than juice.

Oregano Oil has been shown to slow the growth of E. Coli and other bacteria that cause UTI's. The antibacterial compound in Oregano Oil is Carvacol. It is a natural antibiotic that is used to fight common infections. Add Oregano Oil to your diet to prevent UTI's.

Baking Soda & Apple Cider Vinegar is a popular home remedy for UTI's. The combination acidifies the urine that stops bacteria from growing. Mix both together in warm water and drink the solution 3-4 times a day.

Cream of Tartar is an acid salt used for baking and cooking. It is also used as home remedy for UTI's. Add a teaspoon of COT to a cup of warm water or orange juice. Drink twice daily for 5 days. Do not take it for more than 5 days as it has laxative effects and can cause gastrointestinal discomfort.

Corn Silk comes from the silky threads that grow on corn cobs. In traditional Indian medicine, it has been used to treat UTI's and its symptoms. Corn silk comes in a pill or powder form. It is recommended to take 500 mg 2-3 times a day.

Vitamin C in large doses can stop the growth of bacteria by making the urine acidic. Vitamin C supplements are best to take for treatment and prevention.

D-Mannose is a type of sugar found in some fruits. D-Mannose treats UTI's by sticking to the bacteria and flushing it from the bladder during urination. D-Mannose is also found in apples, peaches, oranges and blueberries. Take D-Mannose at the onset of symptoms and you will not need antibiotics. If you have diabetes, check with a medical professional before using.

Probiotics can prevent UTI's due to the naturally occurring good bacteria lactobacilli. Lactobacilli are a part of a normal healthy yoni, however, some women do not produce enough on their own. Lactobacilli kill off E. Coli and stops them from attaching to the cells of the yoni. Probiotics must be taken daily to establish a healthy flora.

Other tips:

Always wash your yoni with a new wash cloth each time you bathe. Bacteria is everywhere - in your shower, counters, and sinks. These bacteria adhere to wet wash cloths after you use them and eventually rub off on your skin once they are used again. This can cause recurrent infections.

Use concentrated Lysol when washing your clothes. This kills 99% of bacteria in your wash. Bacteria can live on your underwear and transfer to your skin if not washed properly.

Change your menstrual pads often. Bacteria love moist wet areas. Also bacteria from your rectum can transfer to your yoni area if pads are kept on too long.

Use an antibacterial like hydrogen peroxide to wipe after having a bowel movement. The main cause of UTI's is bacteria that spreads from the rectum to the yoni. Personal hygiene is the number 1 cause of infection.

HEALTHY GUT FLORA FOR HEALTHY YONI

Your digestive health is vital for the health of your yoni. Lactobacilli is the good bacteria found in your gut that is responsible for maintaining the flora in your vagina. Lactobacilli produce hydrogen peroxide that reduces the colonization of bad pathogens that cause BV, UTI's and other infections like Trichomoniasis. Lactobacilli are also important for establishing a healthy ph balance for your yoni, which controls infections that cause odors. Antibiotic use also kills off good bacteria in the gut, which is why health professionals often recommend eating yogurt while under antibiotic therapy. Yeast infections are a normal occurrence for women after antibiotic use due to a disruption in the intestinal/vaginal flora. Lactobacilli should always be replenished after antibiotic use. You can take probiotics to restore good bacteria and consume foods such as Sauerkraut, Kefir, Yogurt and Tempeh.

HEALING YONI ODORS

Every woman is different and unique in her own way. Every woman has a natural fragrance and so does her yoni. It is quite normal to have a subtle smell but a strong odor is cause for concern. When your yoni's ph balance is thrown off, unpleasant odors become dominant. Several factors are involved when odor is present such as infections, hormones, medications, sexual partners and personal hygiene habits.

Douching

Douching is not widely recommended because it disrupts the normal ph and causes imbalances. In certain cases, douching can cause pelvic infections. However, there are times where douching may be appropriate. Many health practitioners recommend yogurt douches to treat and prevent yeast infections. Douching with Hydrogen Peroxide reduces odors by rebalancing the ph and cleansing bad bacteria. Douching with Povidone-Iodine has been shown to inhibit the growth of bad bacteria while replenishing good bacteria. Douching is always a personal choice.

Personal Hygiene Products

Certain soaps, feminine sprays and other products can cause irritation of the yoni as well as change the ph balance that causes odors. Choose natural soaps with no harsh dyes or chemicals such as Castile or Cetaphil Soap.

Diet

Foods with pungent smells can change the natural fragrance of the yoni. Garlic, meats, sardines, processed foods, and junk foods can produce a strong vaginal odor, while fruits such as pineapples, peaches, strawberries and cranberries produce a sweeter smelling yoni.

Sexual Habits

A man's semen has an alkaline ph balance somewhere between 7.2 – 7.8 which can throw off your ph balance after sex. You can yoni steam or rinse with Hydrogen Peroxide after sex to help rebalance your ph. It will also help prevent new infections.

Activated Charcoal

Activated Charcoal is a binding agent. It is able to reach toxins beneath the skin and bring them to them to the surface for removal. Inserting activated charcoal tablets in the yoni can improve odors by removing any dirt, chemicals or bacteria in and beneath the tissues of the yoni.

Other Tips:

- Make sure no infections are present
- Drink plenty of water

- Do a colon cleanse – backed up bowels can produce vaginal odors
- Use an antiperspirant to keep yoni dry
- Use yoni wipes
- Make sure your ph stays at a normal level
- (test your levels with ph strips)

HEALING INFERTILITY

Infertility can be emotional for women who are trying to conceive without success. It can be exhausting and disheartening to experience infertility during childbearing years. Underlying issues within the female ecosystem are usually the cause. Conditions can range from Endometriosis to PCOS and ovulation irregularities. Women who are unable to conceive often resort to expensive fertility treatments which are not always successful. There are natural ways to help a woman conceive:

Serrapeptase is an enzyme produced by silkworms. It breaks down and dissolves scar tissue and reduces inflammation. Serrapeptase has worked for blocked fallopian tubes and excess scar tissue on the uterus.

Xian Cao is a Chinese herb that is used the unblock fallopian tubes by dissolving scar tissue. Use in combination with Serrapeptase for best results.

Yi Mu Cao also called Chinese Motherwort, has been used to increase fertility by stimulating the blood flow to the uterus. It is best used with Xian Cao and Serrapeptase.

Geritol is a liquid multivitamin that some women swear by when it comes to conceiving. Geritol contains Folic Acid which has been shown to increase fertility. Other important vitamins such Iron which is important for healthy ovulation.

Evening Primrose Oil is a natural source of Omega – 6 fatty acids. It improves the quality of your cervical mucus which creates the best environment for semen to move towards the egg.

Chaste berry (Vitex) increases fertility by helping regulate hormones and menstrual cycles. Vitex restores the right balance to help regulate ovulation.

False Unicorn is an herb used for menstruation, menopause, ovarian cysts, and infertility. It also normalizes hormones. It prevents recurrent miscarriages as well. False Unicorn is best taken in tincture form.

Dong Quai is a Chinese herb often called "female ginseng". It is excellent for the uterus as it increases blood flow to the pelvic area. It also balances hormones.

Ashwagandha is an Ayurvedic herb used by healers around the world. It promotes overall health and improves infertility. Ashwagandha regulates hormones, removes toxins from reproductive organs, increases libido and regulates menstrual cycles.

Maca Root is great for fertility due to its ability to regulate the hormones needed to achieve pregnancy.

Red Clover is an herb for overall wellness. It is a blood purifier. It is also known as estrogens twin. Red Clover thickens the lining of the uterus for better chances of implantation of fertilized egg.

HEALING THE FEMALE LIBIDO

Good Yoni is the divinity of a woman. It is love. Love fo the feminine body and the embodiment of all things cre ated. Your yoni is sacred and should only be shared with those who worship and adore you. Sex is healing to your relationships It helps strengthen the bond between lovers. It communicates on a soul level and it creates a world of pleasure beyond the conscious mind.

Good yoni is one that seeks the deepest desires, yearns with excitement, orgasms with love, and connects the soul. If you have lost your sexual desire, there are certain factors to consider such as hormones (low testosterone), medication, mental state, trauma etc. Emotional healing is important in restoring your sexual desires. Love your yoni, pamper your yoni and treat her like the goddess she is. Here are some natural remedies that have been scientifically proven for sexual healing:

Maca Root is known for its ability to increase the sex drive by restoring hormonal imbalances. It also increases physical stamina and endurance. Your yoni will appreciate this plant!

Horny Goat Weed is a plant traditionally used in Chinese Medicine. It increases blood flow to the yoni and it increases yang energy for sexual desire. It will definitely make you horny. HGW is best taken in tincture form for extra potency.

Damiana is an herbal plant used for medicine. It contains arbutine and flavanoids that have therapeutic properties. It has been known as an aphrodisiac. Taken with Horny Goat Weed it is a sexual powerhouse. If you have never "squirt" or ejaculated before, you can easily with this herbal combination.

Hydrilla is a super food plant. It is packed with vitamins and minerals that supports overall energy and stamina. This plant is known to increase and enhance sexual performance.

Mucuna Pruriens is called the magical bean due to its medicinal properties. It is good for those with low sex drive due to diabetic conditions. It is a great for those who want to "get in the mood" due to its mood boosting agent L-dopa.

L-Arginine is an amino acid that increases nitric oxide which helps circulates blood flow to the clitoris and other erogenous zones in the body to increase sexual desire.

Ginseng + Gingko Biloba are both plants that increase blood flow to the yoni. Ginseng and Gingko also increase dopamine which can help increase sexual mood. They are best when taken together.

Rhodiola is an adaptogenic herb used to treat stress and mental exhaustion. It boosts energy levels and increases sex drive by reducing stress.

Sarsaparilla is a plant used for medicine. It is one of the oldest remedies for sexual enhancement. It works by stimulating sexual hormones in the body.

Royal Jelly is a jelly fed to queen bees. It contains a variety of nutrients that nourish the body. It increases testosterone and improves sexual endurance and stamina.

Rose Tea is tea made from dried organic rose petals. Rose invoke beauty, open the heart and evoke the spirit of love. Rose have been a symbol for the yoni since time began! Drink a cup of rose tea before sex for good energy.

Wild Yam Root contains a potent chemical that resembles the female sex hormone. It increases the sex drive and it increases love fluids during sex.

Tribulus is a native plant to Asia. This Chinese herb has been used for ages in treating low libido. Studies have shown significant changes in desire, arousal, lubrication and orgasms when taking this herb.

Aphrodisiac Foods

- Apples
- Strawberries
- Cherries
- Chocolate
- Asparagus
- Oysters – Can be toxic
- Ginger
- Figs
- Coconut
- Watermelon
- Pomegranate
- Sweet Potatoes

Spices for Love

- Cinnamon
- Vanilla

- o Cloves
- o Nutmeg – Can be toxic
- o Cardamom
- o White Pepper
- o Saffron
- o Rosemary
- o Sage
- o Sweet Basil
- o Marjoram
- o Coriander
- o Fennel

YONI STEAMING

Yoni steaming is an ancient practice. It has been practiced by women in different countries over the world for ages. Yoni steaming is basically a spa treatment for your vagina. Herbs are added to a pot of boiling water and put inside a hole in chair. You sit over the chair as the steam cleanses the yoni for 20 – 30 minutes. You can make a home based yoni steam by putting the boiled herbs in a ceramic bowl and place inside of a clean toilet. Use a towel to drape over your lap. Benefits of yoni steaming include:

- Reduces menstrual cramps
- Boosts fertility
- Shrinks fibroids
- Tones the uterus
- Tightens the yoni
- Promotes healing
- Restores ph balance
- Detoxifies female organs
- Treats hemorrhoids
- Reduces vaginal odors
- Treats vaginal infections
- Reduces pain and discomfort
- Heals womb trauma

Herbs used for Yoni Steaming include:

- Motherwort
- Yarrow
- Raspberry Leaf
- Rose Petals
- Calendula
- Rosemary
- Comfrey
- Fenugreek
- Lavender

YONI DETOX PEARLS

Yoni Detox Pearls are small pea-sized tampons filled with natural herbal ingredients. They are designed to be inserted into the yoni for a maximum of 3 days. The ingredients in the pearls assist in cleansing the womb and the yoni by expelling mucus, old blood, dead tissues, dead cells, yeast, infections, blood clots, toxins and fibroids. The ingredients in Yoni Detox Pearls:

- Cnidium – treats bacterial infections, yeast, infertility and increased sex drive
- Stemona – expels parasites, toxins, relieves swelling
- Fructus Kochiae – anti-inflammatory, relieves itching and burning, heals UTI's, removes toxins
- Motherwort – hydrates yoni, reduces blood loss, reduces painful cycles, expels old blood clots
- Rhizoma – expels dead tissues and tumors, removes dead tissues and skin cells
- Borneol – improves circulation in the womb, reduces swelling and excessive bleeding

Yoni Detox Pearls can vary in ingredients. It is important to research all ingredients before selecting a product. You can also make the yoni pearls in your own kitchen by using loose herbs and gauze. Wrap the herbs in the gauze and form in a circle to make a small insert. Tie a piece of string around the top to close.

nsert the tampon and leave the string outside the yoni for re-
rieval.

HERBS FOR FEMININE HEALING

Black Cohosh – menopause symptoms, PMS, menstrual cramps, hot flashes, vaginal dryness, night sweats, irritability

Calendula – inflammation, vaginal infections, BV and yeast wound healing, eczema

Chamomile – healthy hair, lower blood sugar, menstrual pain, sleep and relaxation, digestion, heart health

Cramp Bark – arthritis, back pain, menstrual cramps, menopause, inflammation, muscle relaxant, regulates hormones

Dandelion Root – inflammation, reduces blood sugar, reduce cholesterol, lower blood pressure, digestion, bladder

Echinacea – reduces breast cancer, anxiety, immune system, pain and swelling, skin care

Fennel – cramps, bloating, weight loss, heart health, anti-cancer, increased milk supply, menopause, memory

Fenugreek – heart, digestion, inflammation, weight loss, diabetes, brain health, breastfeeding, anti-aging

Fleabane – heavy menstrual bleeding, UTI's, diuretic, parasites, tumors, swelling

Ginger – nausea, inflammation, arthritis, ovarian cancer, immune system, menstrual pain, libido

Goldenseal – natural antibiotic, UTI's, skin, infections

Hibiscus – blood pressure, liver cleanse, anti-cancer, digestion, menstrual cramps, weight loss, mental health

Hydrangea – UTI's, inflammation, autoimmune disease, kidney stones, parasites, pain

Lavender – anxiety, depression, relaxation, skin, hair, anti-cancer, pain, aromatherapy

Lemon Balm – menstrual cramps, anxiety, stress, improves mood, pain reliever, cold sores

Licorice Root – skin, ulcers, hepatitis, PMS, balance hormones, reduces stress, pain relief

Motherwort – relives tension and stress, promotes menstruation, heart health, improve blood circulation

Myrrh – bacterial infections, tightens skin, oral health, energy, wound healing, stops excessive bleeding

Nettle – pain reliever, treats ulcers, allergies, diabetes, inflammation, heart health

Oat Straw – anxiety, fatigue, libido, diuretic, urinary tract infections, hair, skin, nails

Passionflower – anxiety, depression, insomnia, blood pressure

Peppermint – headaches, menstrual cramps, allergies, infections, energy, weight loss, sleep

Plantain- UTI's, hemorrhoids, bacteria, swelling

Red Clover – menopause, anti-cancer, heart health, blood cleanser, PMS, sexually transmitted infections

Rosemary – pain reliever, stress, circulation, immune system digestion, hair, allergies

Sage – negative energy, immune system, menopause, diabetes cholesterol, memory

Sassafras – Healthy bladder, skin, pain, circulation, immune system

Skullcap – anxiety, insomnia, heart health, bacterial infections menstrual cramps

Slipper Elm – UTI's, sexual infections, hemorrhoids, IBS, parasites

St John's Wort – anxiety, depression, menopause, skin healing

Uva Ursi – shrinks and tightens yoni, bladder infections, interstitial cystitis

Valerian – menopause, anxiety, headaches, insomnia

Vervain – antibacterial, diuretic, muscle relaxer, UTI's, anxiety, depression

White Willow Bark – pain relief, arthritis, weight loss, skin, menstrual pain

Wild Alum Root – heavy menstrual bleeding, wound healing, gastrointestinal disorders

ESSENTIAL OILS FOR FEMININE HEALING

E ssential oils are made from extracting compounds from plants. They are very potent and have therapeutic properties. Essential oils can be added to baths, carrier oils for massaging, placed on the pressure points on the body, rubbed on your stomach for feminine healing, or added to a diffuser. You can also add essential oils to natural soap to make your own Yoni wash. Essential oils for feminine healing:

Clary Sage – headaches, menstrual pain, PMS, menopause

Ylang Ylang – anxiety, stress, sex, relaxation

Jasmine – pain relief, menopause, skin, improves mood

Geranium – fatigue, stress, hormones, tension, PMS

Lavender – stress, anxiety, sleep, relaxation, rejuvenation

Cypress – heavy bleeding, cramps, improves mood

Peppermint – hair growth, colds, allergies, respiratory

Neroli – skin, improves mood, high blood pressure, sleep

Tea Tree – antiseptic, yeast infections, antiviral

Rose – skin, menstrual pain, anxiety, improves mood, love

Orange – improves mood, sleep, allergies, skin, pain

Rosemary – hair growth, pain, immune system, cramps

Lemon – insomnia, improves mood, pain relief, depression

Ginger – appetite, nausea, respiratory, pain relief

YONI BATHS

Rose Bath – Add red and pink rose petals to warm bath water for love, sex, desire and pampering the yoni

Baking Soda & Apple Cider Vinegar Bath – Add a cupful of each to a warm bath to detoxify the body and cleanse the yoni

Lavender Bath – Boil lavender tea and add to bath water for good smelling relaxed yoni

Sea Salt Bath – Add a cupful of sea salt to a warm bath after menses to draw out toxins and old blood from your womb

Tea Bath – Use your favorite tea in a bag, boil and add to bath water for self love

Herbal Bath – Use any combination of loose herbs, add to boiling water, strain and add to bath water for self care

Essential Oil Bath – Use any combination of essential oils to warm bath water for awakening your divine yoni

Milk & Honey Bath – Add coconut milk and honey to warm bath water for soft and sweet yoni

Alkaline Bath – Add lemon and baking soda to your warm bath water for detoxifying your womb and yoni

Oil Bath – Add olive, coconut, jojoba, sweet almond or vitamin e oil to warm bath water for pampering your yoni

Clay Bath – Add Bentonite clay to your warm bath water to detoxify your womb and yoni

Bubble Bath – Add pure castile soap to your warm bath water for luxurious yoni

YONI WIPES

Yoni wipes are used for personal cleansing. They can be taken while traveling to ensure your yoni is fresh throughout the day or they can be used at home. They can be used before and after sex (although I do not recommend using essential oils before sex because they might burn your man's balls ha-ha-ha). Yoni wipes can make you feel invigorated, and rejuvenated down there. They can also prevent infections. The good thing is they are super easy and very affordable to make yourself.

- 1 pack of unscented wipes
- Liquid Castile soap
- Water
- Essential oil of your choice

Place the unscented wipes in a large zip lock bag. Add 2 tablespoons of Liquid Castile soap to 2 cups of water. Add 20 – 30 drops of essential oil. Peppermint oil and Tea Tree oil are popular essential oils for yoni wipes. Turn bag upside down to ensure even distribution of liquids. Yoni wipes are complete. You can divide them up into several zip lock bags to keep at work, at home, in your car or in your purse.

YONI AFFIRMATIONS

I will honor my Yoni.

I will honor my Womb.

I am whole.

My ovaries are healthy.

My sensuality is not a curse.

I trust and love myself.

I create well-being in my life.

I am deeply loved.

I embrace my sexuality.

My hormones are perfectly balanced.

My menstrual cycle is regular.

I will listen to my intuition.

My body is sacred.

I am radiant, beautiful and strong.

I give my body love and respect.

I forgive myself and others.

I claim my feminine power now!

YONI MUDRA

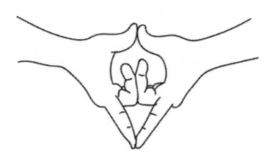

Yoni Mudra is an ancient Indian practice. In Sanskrit, Mudra means "gesture". Mudras are hand positions that help stimulate certain energies in the body. Yoni Mudra is a gesture that promotes a calm state of mind. It represents the "Womb" which is the source of life. Practicing Yoni Mudra brings balance to opposing energies within the body to achieve inner peace. It is designed to detach oneself from the external world and all the tensions associated with it. Yoni Mudra involves meditation. Meditating on healing your Sacral and Root Chakras while practicing Yoni Mudra will greatly improve how you feel about yourself. Your past traumas will begin to heal, your womb will restore itself and you will be able to hear your own voice, your inner goddess. The benefits of Yoni Mudra:

- Balances the central nervous system
- Relaxes the mind
- Spiritual calm
- Self love
- Relieves stress and depression
- Creates inner peace

- Balances Sacral Chakras
- Encourages healing to the womb
- Promotes sacred energy

ABOUT THE AUTHOR

Nikki Love is a Mother of 5, Wellness Coach, Community Herbalist, Yoga Practitioner, Certified Raw Food Chef, Writer, Entrepreneur and Health Enthusiast. She uses many healing modalities such as Reiki, Feng Shui, Pranic Healing, Sound & Music therapy, Crystal Healing, Aromatherapy, Color therapy, Water and Light therapy, Reflexology, and Guided Imagery. Nikki started her natural health journey at the age of 21 when she began to study herbs, homeopathic and alternative medicines. After healing herself from ulcers, gallstones and uterine fibroids she became a self proclaimed healer. Nikki is a lover of nature, healthy food, sunshine, water, good energy and lots of LOVE. She is currently working to release her own line of herbal medicines. Nikki Love is available for private or group wellness sessions. Email Nikkiloveswellness@gmail.com for more information.

Made in the USA
Columbia, SC
31 July 2023

21073624R00040